Achievable Weight Loss Plan

Simon Grier

ISBN: 978-1511983235

DEDICATION

This book is dedicated to everyone that has lost touch with their own ability to maintain a healthy weight.

CONTENTS

ACKNOWLEDGMENTS

I would like to acknowledge my family for their support and encouragement during my own personal weight loss journey.

1 INTROCUTION

Thank you for purchasing the Achievable Weight Loss Plan. This weight loss plan requires no diet products. The Achievable Weight Loss Plan is a system that will enable you to lose weight and then carry on maintaining a healthy weight. As you follow the system you will begin to relearn the healthy eating habits that you were born with.

Note, if you have any special health conditions or dietary needs, please check with your Doctor before proceeding. Firstly I am going to introduce you to some basic facts about weight loss and weight management. You will need to understand these facts to be successful at losing weight. Then, I will expand on each weight loss fact to help you gain a full understanding of each fact and how to apply it to your weight loss journey. Each section has an instruction area, these are the steps you need to follow. Make sure you carry out the instructions and refer back to the explanation for further encouragement. You can step straight in and follow the instructions and read the explanation later if you are really keen to get started. Next, a list of tips and tricks to keep you on your journey. Finally, a meal plan and some additional information. Using my methods, I am convinced you can do it. You are going to look and feel great.

2 BASIC WEIGHT LOSS FACTS

Below are basic facts about weight loss that you need to know. Keep these handy while you are in the weight loss phase.

- Weight Loss is a Numbers Game
- Your Body is a Survival Machine so Successful Weight Loss Requires Hunger Management
- Diet Products and Dieting Hinders Weight Loss
- We Became Overweight because of a Number of Reasons but None of them Matter Now
- You Need to be Kind and Patient With Yourself and Expect to Lose Weight at a Moderate Pace
- You Are going to Feel and Look Amazing

3 MAIN COMPONENTS OF WEIGHT LOSS

Weight Loss Has Two Main Components, that once managed, lead you to a healthy weight.

1. Physical Component - Calories Burnt vs Calories Eaten - science will take care of this
2. Mental Component - Feelings of Hunger, Boredom and Bad Habits - this is where I can help

We will discuss the physical component and then most importantly, the mental component. After you have begun to lose weight you will start to manage these two components naturally without much effort but, at the beginning you need to concentrate on both components and not lose sight of the fact that you are going to look and feel great.

Physical Component

Weight Loss is a Numbers Game

Instructions

*   Set a goal to lose approximately 3/4 to 1 Kilogram per week or less – I say 3/4 to 1 Kilogram but as you become accustomed to controlling your appetite you will undoubtedly have the ability to lose the weight faster.
*   Access an online version of a BMI (Body Mass Index) calculator and ascertain your Healthy Weight Range - record it in the table below
*   Weigh yourself now and write down your current weight and the date below
*   Write down your desired weight goal below, according to your BMI range, choose a weight near the upper end of the scale
*   Take your goal weight from your current weight and divide the answer by 1, this is the number of weeks from the current date to your goal achievement date,
*   Example, Female $80 - 65 = 15$, fifteen weeks from 12 of April 2015 is about July 2015

Table 1

	Healthy Weight Range	Current Weight	Goal Weight	Current Date	Goal Achievement Date
Male	70 to 80 Kilograms	97 Kilograms	80 Kilograms	12 April 2015	September 2015
Female	47 - 64 Kilograms	80 Kilograms	65 Kilograms	12 April 2015	July 2015
Yours					

Explanation

You will be aiming to lose around 3/4 to 1 Kilogram per week. An average size male needs to consume 1600 Calories per day to lose around 3/4 to 1 Kilogram per week. A female needs to consume 1400 Calories per day to lose around 3/4 to 1 Kilogram of weight per week. At this rate you will expect to lose around 3 - 4 Kilograms per month. This will quickly add up. In 6 months' time you will have lost around 20 Kilograms. That is a lot of weight, you will feel much better once you aren't burdened with carrying around the extra weight. As an example pick up something that weighs, 5 Kilos and carry it around the room, see how even that amount is a burden to carry. In reality, carrying around extra weight is what you are doing each day that you are overweight. It is not good for your feet, sleeping patterns, general health and has many related diseases such as Type 2 Diabetes.

Mental Component

Successful Weight Loss Requires Hunger Management

Now that you have set your goal, let's discuss hunger management. Remember your body is a survival machine, when you start cutting calories it is going to think that your food source has become scarce and it will try to trick you into overeating to boost your survival time. To combat this you are going to change from having 3 large main meals per day to 3 smaller main meals and 3 or more snacks per day. Your stomach will need around one week to contract from its stretched state that resulted from consuming large meals. During this first week or two you are going to feel hungry but this will diminish greatly by the end of the second week. This is because, when you go from consuming large meals to smaller snack size meals you are going to get a temporary feeling of emptiness in your stomach but your stomach will re-adjust to the new meal sizes and the hungry feeling will diminish greatly. You will be filling a smaller stomach with smaller meals but more often, therefore staving off feelings of hunger.

Instructions

- You will control your hunger by eating more but smaller meals, your aim is to sit within your calorie weight loss amount for the day but not feel hungry. In order to do this we need to make some calculations.
- Total daily weight loss calorie intake is 1600 for a male or 1400 for a female or use the custom row to add more if you have a physical job or lifestyle - there are guides available online
- The table below breaks down the daily intake into each meal and snack
- You are going to aim to eat no more than the total daily intake per day

Table 2

	Daily Total Weight Loss Calorie Intake	Breakfast Calorie Intake	Snack Calorie Intake	Lunch Calorie Intake	Snack Calorie Intake	Dinner Calorie Intake	Extra Snacks
Male	1600	400	100	200	100	600	200
Female	1400	350	100	200	100	550	100
Custom to be used for physically active people							

4 IDENTIFYING THE RIGHT TYPES OF FOOD

Identifying the Right Types of Food to Eat

To assist you during the adjustment period you will need to identify low calorie snacks. You will need to select foods that have some fiber content, 3 grams per 100 or more is ideal but less is still OK. The food types need to be lighter foods rather than dense foods. For example, light, fiber rich foods are popcorn and salad as opposed to a dense, low fiber, calorie rich, food such as chocolate, cake or biscuits. See additional information section for more examples.

Keep these handy and practice them each day.

- Start to read food packaging labels and become aware of the number of calories contained in foods that you eat regularly, such as bread, ice cream, vegetables and meat. Compare the contained calories to the amount of volume a food has.
- Hunger beating tactics - eating fiber rich foods, sucking on hard lollies and drinking lots of water or carbonated water such as soda water provides a feeling of fullness with low calorie intake. Drink tea or coffee to help suppress hunger. These are the strategies you need to employ to keep yourself from feeling hungry. They are crucial and will greatly assist you in fighting the urge to overeat.
- Try to ignore junk food advertising
- For breakfast choose a cereal that has a fiber content of at least 9% - weigh and measure out the amount required to equal the number of calories you have allotted for breakfast - measure by the spoonful onto the scales. Take note of the number of spoonsful and try to stick to this amount for breakfast each day.
- For snacks choose light fiber rich snacks such as popcorn, aim for around 3% fiber content. Using packaged food such as microwave popcorn allows you to save time measuring, etc. Because the calorie content is listed on the box.
- Drink carbonated water such as soda water. Increase your water intake - if you don't want plain water drink soda water, it has the added advantage of filling your stomach with gas which creates a feeling of fullness. You may want to purchase a soda maker so you

have a constant supply close by when you are watching TV. Try not to drink diet drinks because they are very sweet and trick the body into believing it received calories. When your body realizes it didn't it will make you feel very hungry later.

- Give yourself regular flavor treats. Suck on boiled lollies such as butterscotch because they are long lasting, have plenty of flavor. When you take into consideration the amount of flavor and the lasting experience they turn out to be fairly low calorie at around 22 calories per lolly.

5 DIET PRODUCTS AND EXTREME DIETING

We all have a natural ability to control our weight. When we were very young children we knew when we were full. Unfortunately, well-meaning parents insisted that we eat up and finish everything on the plate. This is one of the reasons we started to fall into the trap of over eating. We can return to that childlike state of knowing when we have eaten enough. If you follow my guidelines you will succeed in losing weight and remaining trim.

Diet products are generally loaded with sugar. Sugar burns fast. Sugar gives you a short term energy boost but after your body has burnt off the sugar you are left feeling hungry. Soon, you will be hungrier than before you ate the diet product. Diet products don't help you manage your hunger. You don't need diet products. The supermarket has lots of foods that you will enjoy, are packed with fiber and are calorie light. You don't need any foods that aren't purchasable down at your local supermarket.

Following diets that require you to purchase special items or foods are a waste of your time and effort and inevitably fail because, they are too difficult to follow when leading a normal busy lifestyle. Making do with the foods in your supermarket and following labelling advice will assist you in sticking to your daily calorie intake. By controlling your calorie intake and allowing yourself to eat any range of foods means you are more likely to stick to your calorie allowance when you are busy or eating out and socializing. It is easy, even when you are out dining and are faced with food that you are unsure of but suspect may contain a large amount of calories, just eat less of that food. For example, if you are dining out and ice cream is presented to you, be aware that ice cream contains about 25 calories per tablespoon, you can still have ice cream just be aware of how much you consume.

6 WHY WE BECAME OVERWEIGHT

We all became overweight for a variety of reasons. It may have been because your parents insisted that you finish all the food on your dinner plate or the pantry at home was stacked with high calorie foods and none of the high fiber low calorie foods. Whatever the reasons for becoming overweight were, they don't matter now. It is time to hang up concerns over why you became overweight and time to start changing your ways. As you progress, you will learn the correct foods and amount of food to eat, so as to feel full. It will be like returning to your younger years. Going through this journey of discovery will recondition you to living a new vibrant life that will enable you to maintain a healthy weight.

7 BE PATIENT AND KIND TO YOURSELF

Expect to lose weight at best, around 3/4 to 1 Kilogram per week. Some weeks will be less and some will be more. Don't push your calorie intake too low to begin with. As you progress you are going to find that controlling your calorie intake is getting easier and easier. You will have become used to eating more but smaller meals. Your stomach won't need to be overfull, for you to feel full. By the time you reach your goal weight this will become second nature to you. Ever noticed that trim people don't usually over indulge at meal and dessert times. This is because it is second nature to them. They don't experience the feeling of missing out as you do while you are overweight.

During the initial phase of weight loss you are going to feel a little bit hungry as you adjust to the new calorie intake. This is natural and I will give you techniques that will help you combat it. It is important to be extra kind to yourself during this period. There are things you can do to compensate for the hungry feelings. For example, keeping chores to a minimum, not over exercising, spending time doing hobbies you enjoy and watching TV. Don't buy too many new outfits yet because they aren't going to fit you in a couple of months' time. I insist you keep exercise to a minimum until you have reached your goal weight. Exercise increases your hunger and intensifies hunger pangs, we don't want this during the weight loss phase because you are trying to manage your hunger, intensifying it will not help. If you enjoy day spas, beauty pampering, having your hair done or massages then I suggest you indulge.

Remember; be patient, if you don't lose 3/4 to 1 Kilogram in a week don't panic, it may be just water intake adding the extra weight to the scales, remain confident. This method does work and it must, because of the science behind it. The most important part to look after is your mental state. Stay strong it will and does get much easier as the days and weeks pass. A week, a month, six months, even a year, all seems a long time looking forward but look back six months, how quickly did the last six months pass? Many years have passed and many more will, the sooner you start the sooner you will get there.

You Are Going to Feel and Look Great

You will gain a feeling of relief as the weight starts coming off. Each week you will feel like a burden has been lifted. As your weight reduces you will feel lighter on your feet. You will be able to stand for long periods without getting sore feet. You are going to get a new sense of confidence. You are going to feel amazing. You are going to look great in new clothes. The clothes will look the way they were designed to look.

Now it's time to get busy move onto the Action Plan to get started................

8 ACTION PLAN AND MEAL PLANS

Adjustment Time

During the first few weeks you are going to be busy adjusting to your new eating plan. You are going to be learning how to combat the initial hunger pains you experience as you move away from overeating. Over eating is causing you to be overly hungry, you are experiencing extra hunger pains because of overeating. If being overweight is causing you to experience poor sleep then it will be causing you to overeat as your body tries to increase your energy levels via food. You are going to reduce your Dinner, Lunch and Breakfast meals and add a lot of extra snack meals plus some flavor treats. This is going to combat your hunger pains and get you used to not overeating. In the past you needed to overeat before you felt full. Your definition of feeling full is going to adjust over the next 3 or so weeks. You are not going to need to overeat anymore to feel full. When a hunger pang comes on you are going to be able to access how much you need to eat to fulfil that hunger pang. It may be just a drink of water or carbonated water that is needed to take away the hunger pang or a hard lolly or a small snack such as fibrous fruit or popcorn. You will be able to gauge your requirements naturally, over time. Children do this, you will return to being able to do it as you did when you were a young child. This is the key to weight reduction and maintenance. You will be able to do this on your own. It will occur naturally as you progress. It is an innate part of all of us. Remember, be patient and kind to yourself, this is really important, especially during the weight loss period.

Let's get started...............

Keep This Close by for the First Few Weeks

- Combating hunger is your number one priority - the hunger you are feeling is a result of your body thinking that you are losing your usual source of calories and is trying to get you to store up. It is only temporary, could last a few weeks but will ease. Eventually you will have full control, recognizing how much food or drink you need to satisfy the hunger you are feeling.
  - Use hunger combat techniques
    - Soda water to fill the stomach with water and gas
    - Low calorie snacks such as popcorn or fibrous fruit such as orange - not fruit juice as it is too high in calories - read food labels select low sugar light foods
    - Between snacks suck on hard lollies, they take a long time to finish and give you a flavor treat - Your body needs flavor treats from time to time, sweet, salty or sour
    - Have one of your snack allowances even if it isn't time
    - Check your watch and see if you can hold on until the next snack time
- If you do any exercise only do low intensity exercise such as a 30 minute walk - exercise will increase your hunger - wait until you reach your weight goal before increasing your daily exercise
- If you don't meet your weight loss target for the week you must get back to your daily weight loss intake and not get worried about it - remember you need to be extra kind to yourself
- Bored, or feeling low, don't eat - watch some TV, drink some Soda Water, suck on a hard lolly, get a haircut, get a massage, get a beauty treatment, go to the shops and look at the clothes you will be buying when you reach your target
- Remember how good you are going to feel and look
- If the journey seems long just take it one hunger pang at a time and think back to how fast time goes
- Believe me when I tell you that you are going to start feeling wonderful, because you are
- Try not to weigh yourself too often, only a couple of times a week so that you aren't put off by weight fluctuations caused by fluid levels or a day that you went over your daily intake level. Remember motivation is very important.

Weight Reduction Meal Plan

- Now that you have worked out the date you expect to reach your weight goal, you have some idea as to how long you are going to have to remain on the weight reduction meal plan. Enter your goal weight and goal achievement date in the table on the next page.

Meals	Male Calories	Female Calories	Custom - to be used for physically active people
Breakfast	400	300	
Beverage or Small Snack	50	50	
Snack	100	100	
Beverage or Small Snack	50	50	
Lunch	200	200	
Snack	100	100	
Beverage or Small Snack	50	50	
Treat	25	25	
Dinner	600	500	
Treat	25	25	
Daily Total Weight Loss Calorie	1600	1400	
Your Goal Weight from Table 1			
Your Goal Weight Achievement Date from Table 1			

Meal Plan

You need to stick to your meal plan until you have reached your goal weight. You can vary the foods being eaten but you must stick to the number of calories allotted to your daily total. To ensure you are getting all the vitamins and minerals you require, include fruit, nuts, legumes, vegetables and meat as per general nutrition advice available on government web sites. You may wish to take a multivitamin during this period, consult with your doctor.

Breakfast

Breakfast - Enter your preferred cereal in the table below. Your breakfast meal needs to contain a high amount of fiber. Remember it should contain at least 9% fiber, this is necessary to prevent excessive hunger during the early part of the day. The fiber burns slower in your body and therefore staves off hunger for longer. Don't choose anything too bland because our body expects a variety of flavors and we shouldn't deprive it of this requirement. Also ensure that the sugar content of the cereal is no higher than 20%, preferably around 15% for cereals that contain fruit, or less for cereals that don't. Too much sugar will cause hunger pangs later. When you eat foods containing high amounts of sugar, your body believes that you have found an amazing source of energy and therefore it will send hunger signals to get you to return to that food source. This also applies to sugar replacements such as stevia or saccharin. Staving off hunger is paramount during the first few weeks because your body is going to attempt to trick you into thinking you are extra hungry during the adjustment period for survival reasons.

- Using scales measure your breakfast weight using a tablespoon - record the number of tablespoons in the table below. You do this to make it easy to get your breakfast ready each morning. Instead of weighing it each morning you can just place the number of tablespoons of cereal into your bowl.
- If you like a beverage with your breakfast record the calories in the table below

	Male Example	Female Example	Yours
Cereal Calories including Milk	350	250	
Tablespoons of Cereal Equal to Cereal Calories	3	2	
Millilitres of milk	100	100	
Beverage Calories		50	
Total Breakfast Calories from Table 3	400	300	

Beverage or Small Snack

	Food and Drink Type	Calories from Table 3
Example	Coffee - 50 Calories	50
Yours		

Snack

- Choosing the right snack is very important. Again, we are concentrating on hunger control. We need to stave off our body's reaction to reduced calories. You need to choose snacks that are low in sugar, have some fiber and are relatively light in composition, popcorn is a good example. Fruit that is relatively low in sugar is also a good choice for snack 1. But, remember high sugar foods make you hungry.

	Snack Calories	Amount of snack, tablespoons or grams etc...	Total allowed snack calories from Table 3
Example	100	Small supermarket microwave packet - 20 grams	100
Yours			

Beverage or Small Snack

	Food and Drink Type	Calories contribute to extra snack calories from Table 3
Example	Coffee and Milk	50
Yours		

Lunch

- Again, choose a convenient low sugar lunch. Perhaps last night's leftovers or a sandwich. Choose something light again. During the weight loss phase it is easier to manage if, once you have worked out the calories for a couple of meals, you repeat those meals rather than preparing different meals each day. Although, if you have the time it is OK to include a variety of meals as long as you are aware or have an approximate idea of the calories being consumed. It is wise to choose something smaller rather than large as you don't want to be uncomfortable for the remainder of your work day. Remember, light in composition, such as salads, is generally light in calories. Don't be too restrictive, this is about managing calories and hunger not fussing over particular food types. You need to keep this as simple and convenient as possible. There are even low calorie choices in fast food restaurants and the calorie content is usually listed.

	Lunch Calories	Amount of Lunch, tablespoons or grams etc...	Total Lunch Calories from Table 3
Example	200	200g Spaghetti Bolognaise from dinner leftovers	200
Yours			

Snack

- Choosing the right snack is very important. Again we are concentrating on hunger control. We need to stave off our body's reaction to reduced calories. You need to choose snacks that are low in sugar, have some fiber and are relatively light in composition, popcorn is a good example. Fruit that is relatively low in sugar is also a good choice for snack 1. But, remember high sugar foods make us hungrier.

	Snack Calories	Amount of snack, tablespoons or grams etc...	Total Snack 2 - from table 3
Example	100	Small supermarket microwave packet - 20 grams	100
Yours			

Beverage or Small Snack

	Food or Drink Types	Calories
Example	Coffee Substitute + Milk	50
Yours		

Beverage or Small Snack

	Food Type	Calories
Example	Butterscotch x 1 + Soda Water	25
Yours		

Dinner

- Again, choose a convenient low sugar Dinner. This meal will most likely be your largest meal of the day but remember you can have a snack later so it isn't your last meal of the day, so no need to make it too large. It is wise to choose something smaller rather than large as you don't want to be uncomfortable at bedtime. Don't be too restrictive, this is about managing calories and hunger not fussing over particular food types. You need to keep this as simple and convenient as possible. If eating out or someone else has prepared the meal remember if it looks dense in composition or has a lot of sugar or fat then just eat a smaller portion size and don't have seconds. Remember, to get your vegetables and fruits throughout the day. Vegetables are generally lower calorie and have much less sugar than fruits so lean more toward vegetables than fruit. Serve your dinner on a small plate rather than a large one.

	Dinner Calories	Serving size, medium sized plate of dinner	Total Dinner - should equal the amount allotted for Dinner
Male Example	600	Salmon and Vegetables	600
Female Example	500	Chicken Fillet and Vegetables	500
Yours			

Beverage or Small Snack

	Hard Lolly's and Soda Water	Calories
Example	Butterscotch x 1	25
Yours		

As You Progress

As the weeks pass you will notice that your weight is dropping off and you are proceeding toward your healthy weight. You will be feeling better, sleeping better and have more energy. Most importantly, you will be starting to recognize which foods are calorie rich and which foods are lower calorie. It will start to become second nature.

Once You Have Reached Your Healthy Weight

By the time you have reached your healthy weight you will have learnt what you need to know to maintain it. You will once again be attuned to your body, like you were when you were a child. There will be no need to calculate calories in a formal manner because you will have the innate ability to recognize calorie rich foods and proportion appropriately. If you want to continue on the meal plan a bit longer adjust the daily calorie intake and meal allowances to 2200 for males and 18000 for females

If you wish to contact me please email me at.
simonachieveableweightloss@gmail.com

See Below for Additional Information.................

9 ADDITIONAL INFORMATION

List of low calorie and low sugar snacks that contain fiber and are quick to make

- Popcorn with small amount of butter and salt
- Salsa on celery or thin wafers
- Carrot sticks, celery or capsicum sticks and hummus
- Baked pita chips
- Parmesan and Rosemary Flatbread Crackers
- Spinach and Feta Dip
- Tomato Turnovers
- There are many more examples with recipes on the internet
- Add your own to this list

Words on food packaging that mean fat or sugar

Fat	Sugar
Vegetable Oil / Fat	Sucrose
Animal Oil / Fat	Maltose
Shortening	Lactose
Lard	Dextrose
Palm Oil	Fructose
Copha	Mannitol
Coconut Oil	Sorbitol
Milk Solids	Xylitol
Monoglycerides	Glucose Syrup
Diglycerides	Corn Syrup
Coconut	Dissacharides
Butter	Honey

Nutrition Claims – What do they really mean?

Reduced Fat: at least 25% less fat than the original product in the same brand but,
The food may still be high in fat.

% Fat free: can only be used for "low fat" product with the percentage based on the weight of fat in 100 grams of food. (In a 100 gram serving of food marked 98% fat free, that serving has 2 grams of fat.)

Cholesterol Free: This does not mean low fat. Cholesterol is only found in food which contains animal fats (only animals make cholesterol – plants do not).
For example, vegetable oils (canola, olive, sunflower etc) are cholesterol free, but are 100% fat.

Light' or 'Lite': This does not necessarily mean low in energy or fat etc. It may mean light in color, lightly toasted, light in salt, light in taste.
No added Sugar:
No added refined sugars. It does not necessarily mean the food is low in sugar, because the food may be high in natural sugars (for example, fruit juices).

'Diet': Usually means artificially sweetened.
Source of fiber:
More than 1g of fiber per 100g
High Fiber: at least 3g of fiber per 100g

Tips, Tricks and What You Need to Know to Achieve and Maintain Your Healthy Weight

Keep this list handy.

- Your body is wired to survive - It sees food as paramount to survival
- Your body will use hunger to control your eating habits and send you back for more high calorie foods such as sugar - the more you have the hungrier you will be
- Losing and maintaining weight is all about controlling hunger, eventually this becomes second nature - this is the key
- Each week your hunger levels will drop dramatically making it easier and easier
- As you search the supermarket and read food labels you will learn which foods tend to fill you, versus others that make you hungry.
    - Foods high in sugar make you hungrier - generally aim to eat foods that contain 10% sugar or less or less than 20% if the food contains fruit such as breakfast cereals.
- Weight Loss Food Facts;
    - Light foods are generally lower calorie
    - Fiber burns slower in your body, staving off hunger
    - Sugar, in its many forms, stimulates your hunger because your body detects it as being good for survival - you need to outsmart your body and tell it who is boss by choosing lower sugar foods. Your hunger will adjust.
    - You need to eat smaller and more times per day when losing weight
    - If you are a fast eater, slow down as it takes 7 minutes for your body to register that you are full.
    - You will eat up to 10 times per day or more as per my plan - this will help you control hunger
    - Thirst can be mistaken for hunger, try a drink between meals before eating
    - Poor sleep makes you hungry, as you lose weight you will sleep better

- You must, be patient with your progress while losing weight - expect to lose up to 3/4 to 1 Kilogram per week, no more
- Be kind to yourself - massages, beauty therapy, relaxation such as reading or watching TV, take it easy until you reach your goal weight
- Breakfast cereals and starchy foods stimulate serotonin which improves your mood - don't exclude these food groups, we are only concerned with reduced calories not excluding food types
- Meats, nuts and proteins stimulate your dopamine which also improves your mood
- Don't carry out vigorous exercise until you have reached your healthy weight because it will make you overly hungry- take it easy, do some light walking only
- Weigh yourself weekly and be proud of your achievements -
    o If you have a week without much weight loss don't get dejected just go straight back into the program it will only delay your progress by one week
- As the weeks and months go by you are going to start feeling much better
    o less hungry and happier
    o less tired and sleeping better
    o lighter on your feet
    o Improved self-image

FINAL NOTE

The journey forward to your healthy weight might feel long but just look back and think about how quickly the past 3, 6 or 12 months has passed.